*N*atural *W*arriors

By

Lori
"the Herbchick"
Osterloh Hagaman

Contents

Appendix

Introduction

We live in an age where the human immune system is continuously bombarded by ever prevalent invaders. It would seem the people around us either have immune systems that either cannot cope or overcompensate. We have been over-treated by antibiotic pharmaceuticals, partly because of the giant companies pushing them and partly because of our laziness in wanting a quick fix. We have enabled various strains of bacteria to run rampant and build up defenses against these medications.

What started as a godsend in the 1940s with the use of penicillin for widespread, bacterial infections has become overly used and abused. Medical professionals walk a fine line when deciding how to treat illnesses. They are burdened with so many factors. They are educated in the best way possible, but yet, things have happened – bacteria have evolved – and we are now faced with new issues. Antibiotic treatments can save lives. Knowing when to use them is an art.

Our agricultural models have allowed antibiotics to enter our food supply via meats. Yes, while there is a holding time for a lot of antibiotic-treated animals before slaughter, there is not one for all of them. Large-scale, factory farms have made the feeding of antibiotics common practice, as a means of preventing various illnesses prevalent in close quarters experienced in the enclosed, factory farm models.
(https://www.ncbi.nlm.nih.gov/pmc/articles/PMC4378521/, accessed 2/23/2017)

As a result, we have bacteria strains that are classified as "superbugs." They are resistant to antibiotics. They require increasingly stronger and stronger antibiotics for treatment, due to the human immune system not being able to handle the increased potency. A 2013 report from the Centers for Disease Control states the following: "Each year in the United States, at least 2 million people become infected with bacteria that are resistant to antibiotics and at least 23,000 people die each year as a direct result of these infections. Many more people die from other conditions that were complicated by an antibiotic-resistant infection" (from https://www.cdc.gov/drugresistance/threat-report-2013/, accessed 2/23/2017)

I decided to write this book **not** as a "cure all." *I believe there is no one cure or solution for every person's ills*. Instead, I intend it as a tool to aid in the building of health. The medical professional community finally realizes the need to avoid antibiotics for non-bacterial infections, and to encourage people to allow their own, natural immune systems to work before rushing in for pharmaceuticals. They have increased the public's awareness of viral infections and how antibiotics are useless, possibly adding harm, against viral and fungal infections. I feel it is essential to have more resources with information on those naturally occurring plants and substances that can enhance our abilities to fight disease.

This book presents my "top ten" list of immune boosters. It is by no means an exhaustive list of those natural substances which may help to promote health or boost immune system function. It is merely the top ten items I go to first when looking to build fitness in this area.

Let's face it, antibiotic pharmaceuticals work. They kill bacteria. Their use has saved countless lives and advanced modern medicine further than previously thought possible. No one knew these tiny microorganisms would develop immunity of their own. No one intended for it to happen. It just has. It is time to recognize the value of the old ways, backed by extensive recent research and studies, can be combined with modern techniques to come up with the best solutions for every individual as needed. It is not a natural vs. modern kind of environment anymore. It just can't be. The medical doctors must join together with the naturalists and herbalist (and visa versa) to put the common good at the forefront. Collectively, much progress and healing can be had.

That being said, I am not a medical doctor. I do not practice medicine. Any information contained in this book is meant for **self-help purposes only.** Should a medical concern arise, I urge you to consult with your medical professional. Always inform your medical professionals of any and all supplements you may be using, as well as any and all pharmaceuticals, both prescription and/or over the counter, you may be using.

CONTRAINDICATIONS:

*A*nd then there is the flip-side of the coin: those individuals who have extreme over-reactions to very minute amounts of toxins, bacteria, viruses, etc. These people become "the boy in the bubble," as they cannot survive the immune responses their own body produces in response to things like their own histamine. These people experience auto-immune-like symptoms.

I have done my best to indicate if a substance stimulates the body's immune responses. **DO NOT** USE SUBSTANCES WHICH STIMULATE THE IMMUNE SYSTEM IF YOU ARE EXPERIENCING AUTO-IMMUNE SYMPTOMS OR IF YOU HAVE BEEN DIAGNOSED WITH AN AUTO-IMMUNE DISORDER/DISEASE BY YOUR MEDICAL PROFESSIONAL! The last thing I intend is to exacerbate an existing disease/disorder. Please, please be wary of this factor and pay attention to each section regarding this detail. Please err on the side of caution and use the information contained in this work as discussion points with your medical specialist.

GARLIC

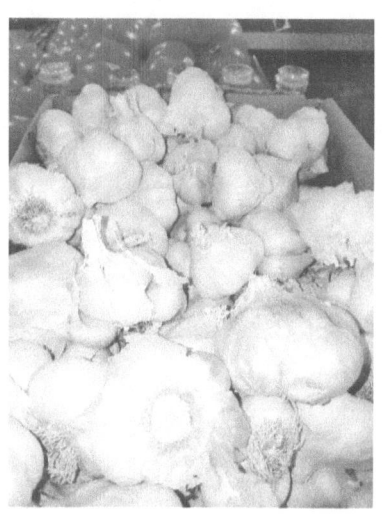

Garlic is a member of the onion family. It is related to leeks and chives, as well. It is thought to have originated in the region of Siberia and spread across the entire globe over 5000 years ago.

Garlic contains a high sulfur compound called allicin, which produces its tell-tale scent. It is a dense nutrient plant. Garlic contains manganese, vitamin B6, vitamin C, and selenium. It also includes calcium, copper, potassium, phosphorus and vitamin B1, all packed with a relatively high amount of fiber, and relatively low calories.

A long history of the traditional medicinal use of garlic exists. It has been written about extensively in the ancient Egypt, India and China. While it has much evidence of its benefits for the circulatory system, I want to draw attention to its value to the immune system.

In one study people were given garlic supplements and compared to a group given a placebo. The group receiving the garlic showed a decrease in the number of days in which the participants felt ill with common cold symptoms. Another study showed that high dosages of a garlic extract supplement (2.56 grams per day) reduced the number of sick days attributed to the cold and flu by 61%. This is thought to do with the increased immune cell proliferation in the group taking the supplement. In short, this means they observed higher numbers of T-cells and NK cells (the cells the human immune system makes to kill foreign invaders).

This is promising research. What is even more encouraging is the newest research showing garlic's ability to enhance the bactericidal effects of pharmaceutical antibiotics against otherwise antibiotic-resistant strains of MRSA and C. albicans (that's "candida", folks). The study I found was in-vitro, meaning it was done in a lab test tube or petri dish, or some similar method (studies done in living subjects is called in vivo). This is exciting as this shows the value of natural processes working in tandem with modern medicine.

Stomach ulcers have been found sometimes to be caused by a bacterium called *Helicobacter pylori* (H. pylori). Studies have shown the ingestion of raw garlic helps to decrease the population of this bacteria, which is wonderful news. This same effect was observed against E.coli. Similar results were observed against vancomycin-resistant *Staphylococcus aureus* and group *A. streptococci*.

As a teen, I always seemed to be cursed with extreme swift illnesses. One minute I'd be sleeping through algebra class and the next I'd have purple, swollen tonsils touching and making me sound like a cartoon character with a 103-degree temperature! Garlic was one of the herbs I used to combat these spells. I would start hitting the garlic immediately

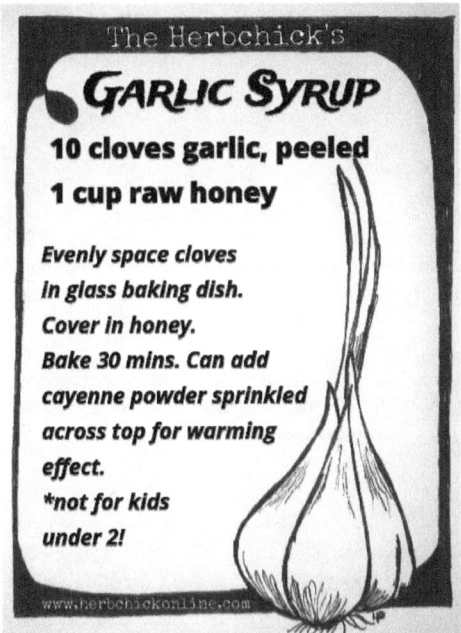

The Herbchick's

GARLIC SYRUP

10 cloves garlic, peeled

1 cup raw honey

Evenly space cloves in glass baking dish.
Cover in honey.
Bake 30 mins. Can add cayenne powder sprinkled across top for warming effect.
*not for kids under 2!

www.herbchickonline.com

when the throat pain would start. I prefer to use garlic oil capsules (sometimes called pearls) – in large quantities. The garlic oil capsules I used were equivalent to 1000 mg of fresh garlic in each little "pearl." I would take five to ten of these per day to deal a death blow to the illness. I also would eat garlic syrup (see illustration) by the spoonful`l and then chase it all down with tea.

It is important to note that I smelled like I had rolled around in an Italian restaurant while consuming these large quantities of garlic. But oozing garlic is not nearly as offensive as some things I could have smelled like. And really, I'd rather feel like a pizza joint than a massive pile of stinky illness.

Sources:

Joe Leech, D. (2017). *11 Proven Health Benefits of Garlic*. [online] Authority Nutrition. Available at: https://authoritynutrition.com/11-proven-health-benefits-of-garlic/ [Accessed 23 Feb. 2017].

Mahmoud Zardast,[1] Kokab Namakin,[2,*] Jamil Esmaelian Kaho,[3] and Sarira Sadat Hashemi[3], (2016). Assessment of antibacterial effect of garlic in patients infected with *Helicobacter pylori* using urease breath test. Avicenna J Phytomed\ v.6(5); Sep-Oct 2016 (accessed 2/23/2017)

Lee, S., Nam, S., Lee, H., Son, S., & Lee, H. (2015). Antibacterial Activity of Aqueous Garlic Extract Against Escherichia coli O157:H7, Salmonella typhimurium and Staphylococcus aureus. *Journal of Food Hygiene and Safety,30*(2), 210-216. doi:10.13103/jfhs.2015.30.2.210

Arzanlou, M. (2016). Inhibition of streptococcal pyrogenic exotoxin B using allicin from garlic. *Microbial Pathogenesis,93*, 166-171. doi:10.1016/j.micpath.2016.02.010

Olive Leaf

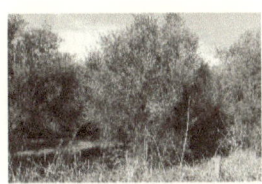Olive Leaf is one of those herbs which might appear to be a panacea when first examined. It does, after all, appear on many sources as a remedy to be used for circulatory system health, similar to garlic. One of its main chemical components, oleuropein, has been shown to combat the formation of new cancer cells in studies and has also been shown to inhibit certain enzymes which create inflammation in some types of arthritis.

It seems Olive Leaf has a historical medicinal use dating back to Ancient Egypt. In Morocco, a tea made from Olive leaves is used for cold-and-flu-like symptoms. There have been many studies, in laboratory settings, which show its promise against certain types of bacteria and viruses, including two kinds of

Staph, the kind which has been found to be resistant to pharmaceutical antibiotic treatment. I am still looking, but free-system data from tests run on real, live people have not been located. However, as I said, I am looking and hoping to find some soon. There are plenty clinical studies with exciting data for its use in decreasing gout acids; lowering harmful blood serum cholesterol levels; and more. I feel confident the promising laboratory research will soon graduate to human trials.

While the Moroccan tea does sound tasty, and I may be adding it to my routine, the easiest way to incorporate olive leaf extract to your regimen is through extracts and capsules. Many offer standardized amount of oleuropein. This is the phenol found in Olive Leaf Extract. I will just say that while it does appear to be the principal operating constituent of the plant, it has been shown to work more efficiently as a whole herb. If it were me, I would want to utilize a product standardized with 50 mg oleuropein, plus the other ingredients found in the extract.

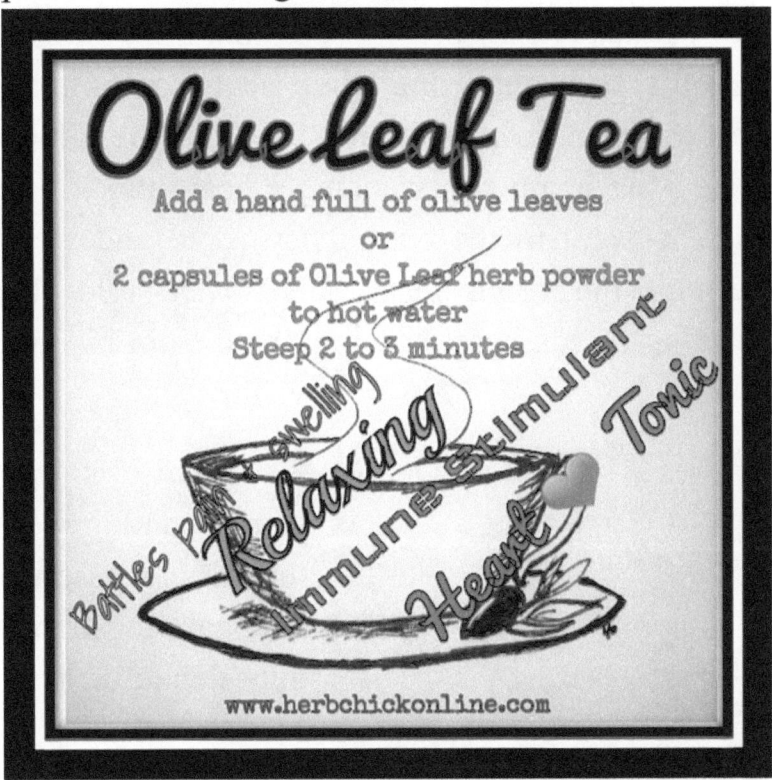

Those who have been in the natural health business have heard of something known as a "healing crisis." This is the idea that a person must go back through the symptoms of the illness for some brief period. While it is out for debate if this is a real phenomenon or not, I want to share a story with you. A gentleman who has been an herbalist for years had suffered many heart attacks (his words) throughout the years. In his 60's, he began using Olive Leaf Extract in an encapsulated form. Within a few days, he felt as if he were again experiencing a heart attack. He said he went to the emergency room and went through the usual tests only to be told the scarring on his heart had improved from his last visit.

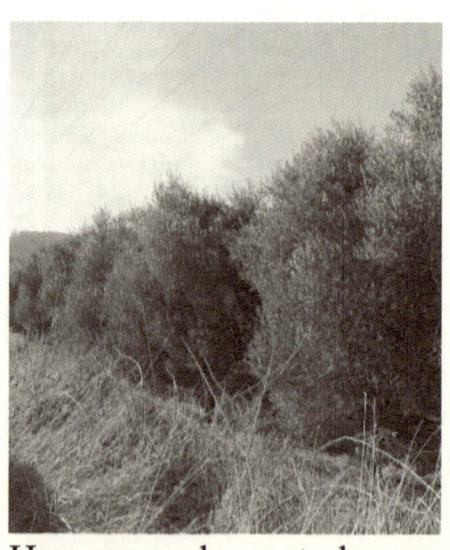

This is his story, and even though some medical personnel may debate it, it is something of which to be aware. **_Never_** disregard heart attack symptoms. However, do not be surprised if you are informed of improvements in your physical conditions with the use of Olive Leaf Extract.

Sources:

OLIVE: Uses, Side Effects, Interactions and Warnings. (n.d.). Retrieved February 25, 2017, from https://www.webmd.com/vitamins-supplements/ingredientmono-233-olive.aspx?activeingredientid=233&activeingredientname=olive

Unexpected Benefits of Olive Leaf Extract. (n.d.). Retrieved February 25, 2017, from http://www.lifeextension.com/Magazine/2013/6/Unexpected-Benefits-of-Olive-Leaf-Extract/Page-01

Babcock, C. (2017, June 21). Olive Leaf Benefits for Cardiovascular Health & Brain Function. Retrieved February 25, 2017, from https://draxe.com/olive-leaf-benefits/

Roxas M, Jurenka J., Colds and influenza: a review of diagnosis and conventional, botanical, and nutritional considerations. Altern Med Rev. 2007 Mar;12(1):25-48.

E. (2017, April 29). Olive leaf extract - Scientific Review on Usage, Dosage, Side Effects. Retrieved February 25, 2017, from https://examine.com/supplements/olive-leaf-extract/

Probiotics

*T*he good bugs. The stuff of life. It has become commonplace for the general public to know replacing the beneficial bacteria in the gut should follow up use of broad spectrum antibiotics. However, there is now research illustrating how probiotics can aid in strengthening the immune system before the use of antibiotics even comes into play.

It has been shown that right, or beneficial, bacteria in the gut may improve the quality of the mucosal membrane in the gastrointestinal tract. This is somewhat to be expected. It has become commonplace, over the last 20 years or so, for medical doctors to suggest the consumption of yogurt containing live and active cultures to their patients using prescription antibiotics. The G.I. health associated with proper beneficial bacteria population is well established and now generally accepted.

New research suggests beneficial bacteria, consumed as supplements, increases non-specific activity of NK cells (an immune system cell). Researchers are recommending supplementation of these probiotics during infancy to head off a host of childhood related illnesses.

The use of probiotics is being associated with decreasing the recovery time from certain immune-related conditions, like upper respiratory infections. Some sources indicate the use of probiotics may hasten the recovery time from antibiotic-resistant infections, like *C.diff* by two thirds.

Sources indicate that the ingestion of multi-strain supplements may be of more significant benefit than single strain supplements. This means getting your probiotics from multiple sources. Not only is it beneficial to use *Lactobacillus acidophilus* and various bifido strains, but many different strains. Examples of those different strains may include *L. Rhamonus*, *L. bulgaricus*, and many more. The count on the number of different strains in the gut was once at about 300. We now know this to be on the conservative side. New figures suggest the name is close to 500, and some research suggests there may be more.

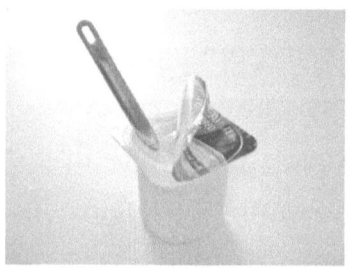 Historically, these bacteria were introduced to the human body upon traveling through the birth canal and via various foodstuff. Dishes such as kefir, fermented fish, sauerkraut, yogurt supplied significant amounts of these good guys. Now, through the advent of sterilization procedures like pasteurization, and even some irradiation procedures, we kill off the majority of these bacteria.

Add in the overuse of prescription antibiotic, antibacterial soap, and the modern fascination of sterilizing every single environment as if it is a surgical room, and you have the recipe for underdeveloped immune systems.

Don't forget that these beneficial bacteria also produce many vitamins that humans require. Vitamin K and some B vitamins are produced by these bacteria. This is one of the easiest ways to boost your immune system. *Lactobacillus* bacterium has even been shown to produce a significant amount of interferon (a signal provided to warn immune cells of the infection of detrimental "germs").

Those who may have a suppressed immune system, please double check with your doctor before use.

Sources:

Dr. Edward Group DC, NP, DACBN, DCBCN, DABFM. (2015, October 14). Research Confirms Probiotics Support Immune System. Retrieved March 2, 2017, from https://www.globalhealingcenter.com/natural-health/research-confirms-probiotics-support-immune-system

Yan, F., & Polk, D. (2011). Probiotics and immune health. *Current Opinion in Gastroenterology, 27*(6), 496-501. doi:10.1097/mog.0b013e32834baa4d

Ashraf, R., & Shah, N. P. (2014). Immune System Stimulation by Probiotic Microorganisms. *Critical Reviews in Food Science and Nutrition,54*(7), 938-956. doi:10.1080/10408398.2011.619671

More Proof That Probiotics Boost Immunity | Prevention. (n.d.). Retrieved from https://www.prevention.com/health/health-concerns/more-proof-probiotics-boost-immunity, retrieved 3/2/2017

Quinteiro-Filho, W., Brisbin, J., Hodgins, D., & Sharif, S. (2015). Lactobacillus and Lactobacillus cell-free culture supernatants modulate chicken macrophage activities. *Research in Veterinary Science, 103,* 170-175. doi:10.1016/j.rvsc.2015.10.005

Jiang, Y., Yang, G., Meng, F., Yang, W., Hu, J., Ye, L., ... Wang, C. (2016). Immunological mechanisms involved in probiotic-mediated protection against Citrobacter rodentium-induced colitis. *Beneficial Microbes, 7*(3), 397-407. doi:10.3920/bm2015.0119

Jiang, Y., Yang, G., Meng, F., Yang, W., Hu, J., Ye, L., ... Wang, C. (2016). Immunological mechanisms involved in probiotic-mediated protection against Citrobacter rodentium-induced colitis. *Beneficial Microbes, 7*(3), 397-407. doi:10.3920/bm2015.0119

http://www.livescience.com/3092-human-gut-loaded-bacteria-thought.html, accessed 3/2/2017

Morelli, L. (2017). Bacteria in Yogurt and Strain-Dependent Effects on Gut Health. *Yogurt in Health and Disease Prevention*, 395-410. doi:10.1016/b978-0-12-805134-4.00023-7

The Importance of Good Bacteria for Health (Stinking Gut). (n.d.). Retrieved from https://wellnessmama.com/2303/stinking-gut/, accessed 3/2/2017

The Top Probiotics For Digestive Health -- Barron Report. (n.d.). Retrieved from https://jonbarron.org/article/probiotic-miracle, accessed 3/2/2017

Frøkiær, H., Henningsen, L., Metzdorff, S. B., Weiss, G., Roller, M., Flanagan, J., ... Ibarra, A. (2012). Astragalus Root and Elderberry Fruit Extracts Enhance the IFN-β Stimulatory Effects of Lactobacillus acidophilus in Murine-Derived Dendritic Cells. *PLoS ONE, 7*(10), e47878. doi:10.1371/journal.pone.0047878,

Photo credit:

Lotus head, http://www.freeimages.com/photo/yogurt-healthy-snack-1513988, 5/18/2017

Oregano

*G*ood luck and fortune are said to come to those who have oregano growing by their home. If this is true, then I should be reeling in the good vibes! I have a large perennial bush of this in my garden.

This native of Europe and central Asia was long used as a medicine before it was a

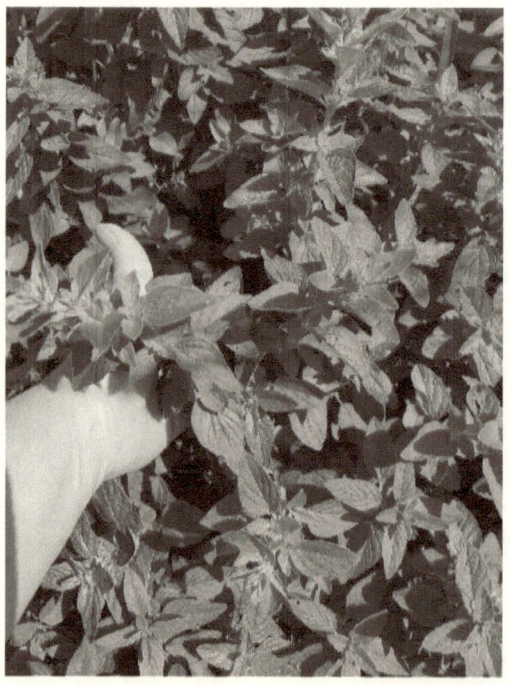 flavorful food additive. It is said to be a gift of the goddess Aphrodite in Greek classics, and its name translates to love of the mountains. Sometimes referred to as "sweet

marjoram," it is used in many dishes, mainly Italian ones. It was widely adopted in the western hemisphere and can be found in many Mexican dishes, as well.

The plant grows in a bush-like a manner and can become quite invasive. I know my oregano patch at home has become a well-established shrub through its underground root system. It can exhibit some inhibitory effects upon neighboring plants. This is something those looking to cultivate it around other food crops and herbs should know and take into consideration.

Most believe oregano found its way to China via the Silk Road. There, it was used by Chinese doctors to relieve fever, vomiting, diarrhea, jaundice, and itchy skin. Extracts of oregano extract have cytotoxic, antioxidant, and antibacterial activities mostly attributed to carvacrol and thymol (active constituents of the plant). It has been investigated for its antifungal effects, making it of particular interest in fighting *Candida albicans*.

Studies in pigs indicate that oregano has a "nonspecific" stimulatory effect on the immune system. Administering oregano to growth stunted hogs resulted in increased immune cell counts. Further studies in this species indicated that the oregano component carvacrol might be the responsible constituent for promoting cell apoptosis (spontaneous cell death) of specific harmful cells.

So how do you use this pizza seasoning to your advantage? Tea is a widespread use. When oregano is steeped in boiling water, it does transfer the taste along with the antimicrobial constituents. While it is highly efficient, it kind of tastes like your sucking down disinfectant water. If that is not a flavor you think you could tolerate, there is the option of encapsulated oregano. This is a more taste bud friendly way of getting therapeutic quantities into your system without having to deal with the disinfectant like taste.

Essential oil of oregano has recently found much acclaim in the natural remedy world. It should be remembered that essential oils are a very concentrated part of plant. Oregano essential oil is no different. It is very potent. Many of the studies I found referred directly to its use in animal and lab experiments. I have only a bit of caution here: I do not ever suggest using Oregano essential oil neat (this is a term in aromatherapy indicating the use of an essential oil without a carrier). A carrier oil or water dilution should always be used so as to not burn the skin or delicate tissues.

Sources:

Oregano. (n.d.). Retrieved from http://www.herballegacy.com/Branca_History.html accessed 3/4/2017

Where did oregano originate? | Reference.com. (n.d.). Retrieved from https://www.reference.com/food/did-oregano-originate-664163b52c658474# accessed 3/4/2017

History of Oregano - InDepthInfo. (n.d.). Retrieved from http://www.indepthinfo.com/oregano/history.shtml, accessed 3/4/2017

The History of Oregano | MySpicer.com | Spices, Herbs & Seasonings. (n.d.). Retrieved from https://www.myspicer.com/history-of-oregano/ accessed 3/4/2017

Melo AD[1], Amaral AF[1], Schaefer G[1], Luciano FB[1], de Andrade C[1], Costa LB[1], Rostagno MH[1] Antimicrobial effect against different bacterial strains and bacterial adaptation to essential oils used as feed additives Can J Vet Res. 2015 Oct;79(4):285-9

Coccimiglio, J., Alipour, M., Jiang, Z., Gottardo, C., & Suntres, Z. (2016). Antioxidant, Antibacterial, and Cytotoxic Activities of the EthanolicOriganum vulgareExtract and Its Major Constituents. *Oxidative Medicine and Cellular Longevity, 2016*, 1-8. doi:10.1155/2016/1404505

Al Hafi, M., El Beyrouthy, M., Ouaini, N., Stien, D., Rutledge, D., & Chaillou, S. (2016). Chemical Composition and Antimicrobial Activity ofOriganum libanoticum,Origanum ehrenbergii, andOriganum syriacumGrowing Wild in Lebanon. *Chemistry & Biodiversity, 13*(5), 555-560. doi:10.1002/cbdv.201500178

Pesavento G, Maggini V, Maida I, Lo Nostro A, Calonico C, Sassoli C, Perrin E, Fondi M, Mengoni A, Chiellini C, Vannacci A, Gallo E, Gori L, Bogani P, Bilia AR, Campana S, Ravenni N, Dolce D, Firenzuoli F, Fani R (2016) Essential Oil from Origanum vulgare Completely Inhibits the Growth of Multidrug-Resistant Cystic Fibrosis Pathogens.*Nat Prod Commun.* 2016 Jun;11(6):861-4.

Harmati M[1], Gyukity-Sebestyen E[1], Dobra G[1], Terhes G[2], Urban E[2], Decsi G[3], Mimica-Dukić N[4], Lesjak M[4], Simin N[4], Pap B[5], Nemeth IB[6], Buzas K[1,3].(2017) A binary mixture of Satureja hortensis and Origanum vulgare subsp. hirtum essential oils: in vivo therapeutic efficiency against Helicobacter pylori infection. *Helicobacter.* 2017 Apr;22(2). doi: 10.1111/hel.12350. Epub 2016 Aug 31

Polat, R., & Satıl, F. (2012). An ethnobotanical survey of medicinal plants in Edremit Gulf (Balıkesir – Turkey). *Journal of Ethnopharmacology, 139*(2), 626-641. doi:10.1016/j.jep.2011.12.004

Gómez-Estrada, H., Díaz-Castillo, F., Franco-Ospina, L., Mercado-Camargo, J., Guzmán-Ledezma, J., Medina, J., & Gaitán-Ibarra, R. (2011). Folk medicine in the northern coast of Colombia: an overview. *Journal of Ethnobiology and Ethnomedicine, 7*(1), 27. doi:10.1186/1746-4269-7-27

Walter BM[1], Bilkei G. (2004) Immunostimulatory effect of dietary oregano etheric oils on lymphocytes from growth-retarded, low-weight growing-finishing pigs and productivity.Tijdschr Diergeneeskd. 2004 Mar 15;129(6):178-81

Bimczok, D., Rau, H., Sewekow, E., Janczyk, P., Souffrant, W. B., & Rothkötter, H. (2008). Influence of carvacrol on proliferation and survival of porcine lymphocytes and intestinal epithelial cells in vitro. *Toxicology in Vitro, 22*(3), 652-658. doi:10.1016/j.tiv.2007.11.023

28

Paul, I., Balstad, T. R., Kolberg, M., Pedersen, M. K., Austenaa, L. M., Jacobs, D. R., & Blomhoff, R. (2010). Extract of Oregano, Coffee, Thyme, Clove, and Walnuts Inhibits NF- B in Monocytes and in Transgenic Reporter Mice. *Cancer Prevention Research, 3*(5), 653-663. doi:10.1158/1940-6207.capr-09-0089

Stelter, K., Frahm, J., Paulsen, J., Berk, A., Kleinwächter, M., Selmar, D., & Dänicke, S. (2013). Effects of oregano on performance and immunomodulating factors in weaned piglets. *Archives of Animal Nutrition, 67*(6), 461-476. doi:10.1080/1745039x.2013.858897

Thyme

*O*nce a component of the Egyptian mummification process, Thyme has a long and extensive medicinal history. The Greeks used it as incense in their temples and added it to their baths. The Germans used it in cheese making and brewing procedures. Hippocrates recommended it for use during times of respiratory illness and it was grown in gardens across the country sides. It is said to have even been added to the "posies" worn during the Black Death plagues in the 1300s in Europe (this practice has not been supported by modern research).

Thyme is a classic kitchen herb. Its essential oil was once used as an ingredient in a liquid used to sterilize surgical tools and is still found in Listerine © mouthwash.

Studies show Thyme to be effective against many bacterial and fungal type infections. Many studies indicate it may hold promise for use to aid in the treatment of certain strains of antibiotic-resistant bacterial infections. Thyme has also been shown to be as effective, or more effective than placebos in some studies investigating its use in respiratory illnesses. This has been speculated to be due to its effects on the enzymatic processes producing inflammation. It even has been shown to have a

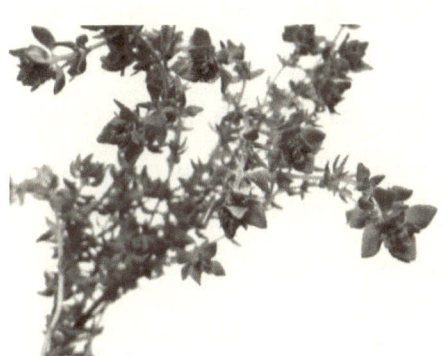 cytotoxic (cell-killing) effect on H460 cancer cells.

Thyme is another herb that possesses a very medicine-y taste. I know that I am not crazy about sucking down a cupful of disinfectant tasting tea. I prefer to use Thyme in encapsulated formulas when consuming it internally. It can make a person nauseated, though. Therefore, if a person is going to take thyme capsules, it is probably best to consume them with a bit of food to not irritate the stomach.

Another way to exploit the antimicrobial aspects of Thyme is by using the essential oil. While I never advocate the internal consumption of essential oils, it is can be useful to diffuse the essential oil. It can be added, in small amounts (I'm talking like five to ten drops) in a bathtub of water. This opens the pores and promotes sweating. Do be aware: Thyme is in the mint family and contains menthols. This means it will increase the sensation of heat or cold if added to the bath water and applied to the skin. It can make the skin more susceptible to temperature burns. It is a good idea to dial down the bath water temperature to avoid this happening to you.

Sources:

Schönknecht K[1], Krauss H[2], Jambor J[3], Fal AM[4]. Treatment of cough in respiratory tract infections - the effect of combining the natural active compounds with thymol (2016) Wiad Lek. 2016;69(6):791-798, accessed 4/4/2017

Šmejkal K, Rjašková V., Use of plant extracts as an efficient alternative therapy for respiratory tract infections (2016) Ceska Slov Farm. Fall 2016;65(4):139-160; accessed 4/4/2017

Oliviero, M., Romilde, I., Beatrice, M. M., Matteo, V., Giovanna, N., Consuelo, A., ... Massimo, N. (2016). Evaluations of thyme extract effects in human normal bronchial and tracheal epithelial cell lines and in human lung cancer cell line. *Chemico-Biological Interactions, 256*, 125-133. doi: 10.1016/j.cbi.2016.06.024, accessed 4/4/2017

Wagner, Luise, et al. "Herbal Medicine for Cough: a Systematic Review and Meta-Analysis."*Forschende KomplementÃ¤Rmedizin / Research in Complementary Medicine*, vol. 22, no. 6, 2015, pp. 359–368., doi:10.1159/000442111, accessed 4/4/2017

Sakkas, H., & Papadopoulou, C. (2017). Antimicrobial Activity of Basil, Oregano, and Thyme Essential Oils. *Journal of Microbiology and Biotechnology, 27*(3), 429-438. doi:10.4014/jmb.1608.08024, accessed 4/4/2017

Mandras, N., Nostro, A., Roana, J., Scalas, D., Banche, G., Ghisetti, V., ... Tullio, V. (2016). Liquid and vapour-phase antifungal activities of essential oils against Candida albicans and non-albicans Candida. *BMC Complementary and Alternative Medicine, 16*(1). doi:10.1186/s12906-016-1316-5, accessed 4/4/2017

Sánchez, G., & Aznar, R. (2015). Evaluation of Natural Compounds of Plant Origin for Inactivation of Enteric Viruses. *Food and Environmental Virology, 7*(2), 183-187. doi:10.1007/s12560-015-9181-9, accessed 4/4/2017

What are the Health Benefits of Thyme? (n.d.). Retrieved from https://www.medicalnewstoday.com/articles/266016.php, accessed 4/4/2017

photo credit:

Zsuzsa, N. K.Retrieved from http://www.freeimages.com/photo/thyme-1321404, 5/18/2017

Golden Seal

Golden Seal is often found in remedies with Echinacea (next section). They are usually thought of as a dynamic duo for the immune system. It was once found growing wild throughout the greater Ohio Valley region, from Ohio to Missouri and from Ontario to Georgia. It is now just one variety of endangered plant being encouraged throughout that region by organizations like United Plant Savers. This buttercup relative is a Native American remedy for inflammatory conditions, like skin rashes.

Golden Seal is very high in a component called berberine. It is this component which helps to give Golden Seal root its characteristic yellow-gold color. Recent studies point to berberine's abilities to behave as an antifungal agent as well as a pretty powerful antioxidant. While it does not seem to have a direct effect on the function or quantity of the immune cells, it seems to keep inflammation (swelling) in check. It has been shown to have a beneficial effect on

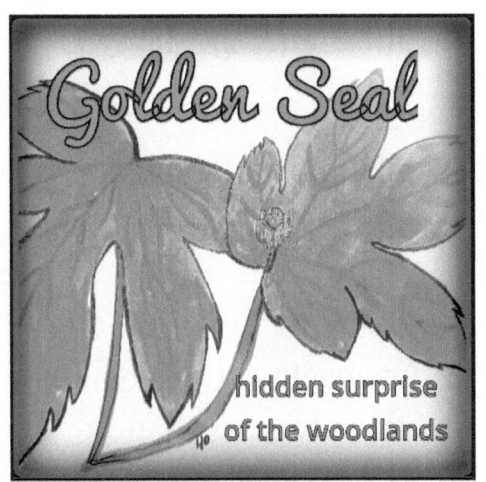

Golden Seal

hidden surprise
of the woodlands

inflammatory conditions, such as sore throats during respiratory infections. It also can stimulate the flow of various digestive juices, like hydrochloric acid. This flow of digestive fluids has immune system benefits, as well. It is usually suggested to use Golden Seal for ailments of the upper respiratory tract, which manifest with hot, swollen traits. This would be like swollen, sore throats. Berberine increases the health of the vascular system. It is thought this attribute enables the strengthening of the tiny blood vessels just below the layers of the mucous membranes in the respiratory system and increases the flow of lymph. This is thought to help spur healing and the body's return to health.

Commonly, Golden Seal is available in health food stores as a bright yellow powder. Occasionally, I have found pieces of the root, but not often. Golden Seal root is bitter. Not a little bitter, but downright acrid. My mother used to say, "that stuff tastes like battery acid." Its taste draws saliva from your mouth upon impact. It is this bitter taste that gets the digestive juices flowing. It is also the reason why tinctures and extracts containing Golden Seal taste "God-awful" to some people. So, while I like to use the tincture for an immediate action, some people may not be able to tolerate the taste. That person might prefer to use Golden Seal in an encapsulated form, by itself or in combination with other immune boosters (such as echinacea, for one example).

**NOTE: some sources indicate Golden Seal might have an impact on blood sugar levels. Please be aware of this possible action and keep an eye on your blood sugar levels if you decide to use it. Those medically diagnosed with diabetes (in any form) or hypoglycemia should consult a physician before its use.

Sources:

Echinacea and Goldenseal: The Dynamic Duo – Dr. Christopher Hobbs. (n.d.). Retrieved from http://www.christopherhobbs.com/library/articles-on-herbs-and-health/echinacea-and-goldenseal-the-dynamic-duo /, accessed 4/20/2017

Goldenseal: A Natural Antibiotic & Cancer Fighter - Dr. Axe. (n.d.). Retrieved from https://draxe.com/goldenseal /, accessed 4/20/2017

Is Goldenseal the Cure for Everything? (n.d.). Retrieved from http://www.healthline.com/health/goldenseal-cure-for-everything, accessed 4/20/2017

GOLDENSEAL: Uses, Side Effects, Interactions, and Warnings - WebMD. (n.d.). Retrieved from http://www.webmd.com/vitamins-supplements/ingredientmono-943-goldenseal.aspx?activeingredientid=943&, accessed 4/20/2017

Natures Remedies Ch 14. (n.d.). Retrieved from http://www.homesteadschools.com/nursing/courses/Natures%20Remedies/Ch%2014%20text.htm, accessed 4/20/2017

Health Benefits of Echinacea & Goldenseal. (n.d.). Retrieved from http://blog.primohealthcoach.com/echinacea-goldenseal, accessed 4/20/2017

Goldenseal | University of Maryland Medical Center. (n.d.). Retrieved from http://www.umm.edu/health/medical/altmed/herb/goldenseal, accessed 4/20/2017

http://www.herbchickonline.com/berberine-a-golden-health-nugget/, accessed 4/20/2017

Rehman, J., Dillow, J. M., Carter, S. M., Chou, J., Le, B., & Maisel, A. S. (1999). Increased production of antigen-specific immunoglobulins G and M following in vivo treatment with the medicinal plants Echinacea Angustifolia and Hydrastis Canadensis. *Immunology Letters, 68*(2-3), 391-395. doi:10.1016/s0165-2478(99)00085-1, accessed 4/20/2017

Clement-Kruzel, S., Hwang, S., Kruzel, M. C., Dasgupta, A., & Actor, J. K. (2008). Immune Modulation of Macrophage Pro-Inflammatory Response by Goldenseal andAstragalusExtracts. *Journal of Medicinal Food, 11*(3), 493-498. doi:10.1089/jmf.2008.0044, accessed 4/2017

Guidotti, A. M., Cunha, B. G., Paulini, M. B., Goiato, M. C., Dos Santos, D. M., Duque, C., ... Gottardo de Almeida, M. T. (2016). Antimicrobial activity of conventional and plant-extract disinfectant solutions on microbial biofilms on a maxillofacial polymer surface. *The Journal of Prosthetic Dentistry, 116*(1), 136-143. doi:10.1016/j.prosdent.2015.12.014, accessed 4/20/2017

Da Silva, A. R., De Andrade Neto, J. B., Da Silva, C. R., Campos, R. D., Costa Silva, R. A., Freitas, D. D., ... Nobre Júnior, H. V. (2016). Berberine Antifungal Activity in Fluconazole-Resistant Pathogenic Yeasts: Action Mechanism Evaluated by Flow Cytometry and Biofilm Growth Inhibition in Candida spp. *Antimicrobial Agents and Chemotherapy, 60*(6), 3551-3557. doi:10.1128/aac.01846-15, accessed 4/20/2017

Habtemariam, S. (2016). Berberine and inflammatory bowel disease: A concise review. *Pharmacological Research, 113*, 592-599. doi:10.1016/j.phrs.2016.09.041, accessed 4/20/2017

Cicero, A. F., & Baggioni, A. (2016). Berberine and Its Role in Chronic Disease. *Advances in Experimental Medicine and Biology*, 27-45. doi:10.1007/978-3-319-41334-1_2, accessed 4/20/2017

Echinacea

*T*he prairies of the United States are home to one of the most popular immune boosting plants on the green market today. Echinacea is commonly called purple coneflower and can be found growing in the

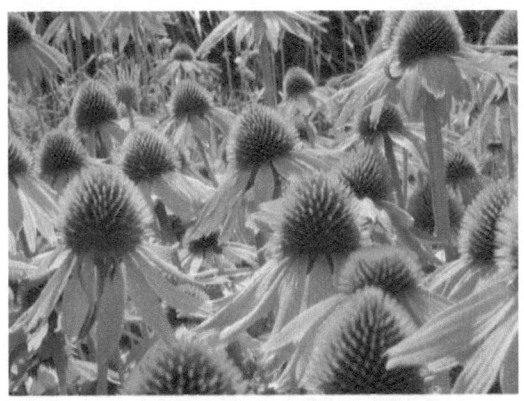

grasslands as a wildflower. There are many species and varieties of Echinacea; however, *Echinacea purpurea* is the one found in most studies.

This plant features a purple to lavender colored daisy-like flower. The center of the flower is usually considerably raised, giving it the illusion of having a cone in the middle.

Echinacea has been found in studies to have an immune-stimulatory effect. It seems to kick T cells into high gear. Interferon, a substance immune cells make as a warning signal to other immune cells, increases when Echinacea is used.

The root contains polysaccharides, glycoproteins, alkamides, volatile oils, and flavonoids which work to stimulate the production of new T-cells and killer lymphocytes.

Even though the above has been indicated by studies, other research fails to show the use of this herb to be of any benefit once you have become ill with the common cold. Some research indicates the real interest may come from utilizing it before actually becoming ill. Even then, there is no research indicating long-term safety of use.

It should be noted some children, as part of an allergic reaction, have broken out in rashes. While it is possible to experience an allergic reaction to any substance, plant materials must be watched closely in the event of an allergic reaction when used. I have seen some clients use this herb and go through Hay Fever-like symptoms. The risk of allergic reaction is what keeps Echinacea on my honorable mention list, as far as immune stimulants go. Some people swear by it. I remain skeptical of this one.

In the occasions I have used Echinacea, the best outcomes have occurred when it is blended with Golden Seal. These two seem to have a dynamic duo effect. In my opinion, each seems to work better when combined with the other. As always, pay attention to the counterindications of both!

Those who have been diagnosed with tuberculosis, leukemia, diabetes, connective tissue disorders, multiple sclerosis, HIV or AIDS, any autoimmune diseases, or, possibly, liver disorders **should not take Echinacea. There also is possible concern about it being used by those making immunosuppressant prescription medications (example: organ transplant recipients and those with specific autoimmune disorders).

Sources:

Echinacea purpurea Benefits & Information. (n.d.). Retrieved from http://www.herbwisdom.com/herb-echinacea.html, accessed 4/20/2017

Echinacea and Goldenseal: The Dynamic Duo – Dr. Christopher Hobbs. (n.d.). Retrieved from http://www.christopherhobbs.com/library/articles-on-herbs-and-health/echinacea-and-goldenseal-the-dynamic-duo/accessed 4/20/2017

USDA NRCS National Plant Data Center.Retrieved from https://plants.usda.gov/plantguide/pdf/cs_ecpu.pdf, accessed 4/20/2017

9 Echinacea Benefits from Colds to Cancer - Dr. Axe. (n.d.). Retrieved from https://draxe.com/echinacea-benefits /, accessed 4/20/2017

Echinacea Benefits: A Potent Natural Remedy (+ a Caution!) | Wellness Mama. (n.d.). Retrieved from https://wellnessmama.com/25999/echinacea-benefits-uses/accessed 4/20/2017

Echinacea | University of Maryland Medical Center. (n.d.). Retrieved from http://www.umm.edu/health/medical/altmed/herb/Echinacea, 4/20/2017

Echinacea Tea – Get an Immune System Boost. (n.d.). Retrieved from http://www.therighttea.com/echinacea-tea.html, accessed 4/20/2017

Il'nyts'kyī RI, IMMUNOLOGICAL REACTIVITY AND CORRECTION OF IMMUNOLOGICAL DISORDERS BY BIOLOGICAL MEDICINES IN PATIENTS WITH CHRONIC OBSTRUCTIVE PULMONARY DISEASE EXACERBATIONS (2014) Lik Sprava. Jul-Aug;(7-8):22-7, accessed 4/20/2017

Torkan, S., Khamesipour, F., & Katsande, S. (2015). Evaluating the effect of oral administration ofEchinaceahydroethanolic extract on the immune system in dog. *Autonomic and Autacoid Pharmacology*, *35*(1-2), 9-13. doi:10.1111/aap.12024, accessed 4/20/2017

Schapowal, A., Klein, P., & Johnston, S. L. (2015). Echinacea Reduces the Risk of Recurrent Respiratory Tract Infections and Complications: A Meta-Analysis of Randomized Controlled Trials. *Advances in Therapy*, *32*(3), 187-200. doi:10.1007/s12325-015-0194-4, accessed 4/20/2017

Dapas, B., Dall'Acqua, S., Bulla, R., Agostinis, C., Perissutti, B., Invernizzi, S., ... Voinovich, D. (2014). Immunomodulation mediated by a herbal syrup containing a standardized Echinacea root extract: A pilot study in healthy human subjects on cytokine gene expression. *Phytomedicine*, *21*(11), 1406-1410. doi:10.1016/j.phymed.2014.04.034, accessed 4/20/2017

Immune enhancing effects of Echinacea purpurea root extract by reducing regulatory T cell number and function. - PubMed - NCBI. (n.d.). Retrieved from https://www.ncbi.nlm.nih.gov/pubmed/24868871, accessed 4/20/2017

Natural immunomodulators and their stimulation of immune reaction: true or false? - PubMed - NCBI. (n.d.). Retrieved from https://www.ncbi.nlm.nih.gov/pubmed/24778031, 4/20/2017

Fonseca, F., Papanicolaou, G., Lin, H., Lau, C., Kennelly, E., Cassileth, B., & Cunningham-Rundles, S. (2012). Echinacea Purpurea L. modulates human t-cell cytokine response. *Planta Medica*, *78*(11). doi:10.1055/s-0032-1320440, 4/20/2017

Echinacea | NCCIH. (n.d.). Retrieved from https://nccih.nih.gov/health/echinacea/ataglance.htm#hed5, 5/18/2017

photo credit:

Townsend, G .Retrieved from http://www.freeimages.com/photo/group-of-echinacea-15267715/18/2017

Boneset

*N*orth America is home to many plants the Native Americans found extremely valuable in times of illness. One of these plants is Boneset (*Eupatorium perfoliatum*). This flowering herb is found in wetland areas from Nova Scotia to Florida and from Texas east, mainly in North America. It was listed in the United States Pharmacopeia, but not in similar books in Europe of the same period. It can be found growing in old fields and usually reaches a height of about two to four feet in height but can be as tall as five feet. This member of the sunflower family features white flowers which appear as if they are hairy in that the petals grow in a way that gives it a fuzzy appearance. The leaves are long and serrated.

The traditional uses for Boneset include reducing the pain associated with high fevers and inducing a sweat. These can be quite useful. Its use diminished after aspirin became common.

It has been used in homeopathic preparations. A homeopathic preparation of this herb was found to be just as effective as acetylsalicylic acid in the treatment of the common cold (results determined by patient checklists). Extracts of the plant have shown some antibacterial activity against gram-positive bacteria. *Streptococcus* bacteria are just one example of gram-positive bacteria. However, most of the results of modern scientific studies of Boneset do not show marked results in the way of immune-stimulation. Where it shines is in the department of reducing inflammation. So, while it may not immediately kick your immune cells into action, it can lessen the pain and undesirable effects of your immune system going to work on the bad guys. One study did, however, publish that it worked against the influenza virus by stopping the virus' attachment to the host cells.

It seems smaller amounts of this herb go a long way. BONESET IS CONTRAINDICATED DURING PREGNANCY AND LARGE

AMOUNTS MAY RESULT IN DIARRHEA AND VOMITING.

Sources:

Derksen, A., Kühn, J., Hafezi, W., Sendker, J., Ehrhardt, C., Ludwig, S., & Hensel, A. (2016). Antiviral activity of hydroalcoholic extract from Eupatorium perfoliatum L. against the attachment of influenza A virus. *Journal of Ethnopharmacology, 188*, 144-152. doi:10.1016/j.jep.2016.05.016, accessed 4/21/2017

Hensel, A., Maas, M., Sendker, J., Lechtenberg, M., Petereit, F., Deters, A., ... Stark, T. (2011). Eupatorium perfoliatum L.: Phytochemistry, traditional use, and current applications. *Journal of Ethnopharmacology, 138*(3), 641-651. doi:10.1016/j.jep.2011.10.002, accessed 4/21/2017

Maas, M., Deters, A. M., & Hensel, A. (2011). Anti-inflammatory activity of Eupatorium perfoliatum L. extracts, eupafolin, and dimeric guaianolide via iNOS inhibitory activity and modulation of inflammation-related cytokines and chemokines. *Journal of Ethnopharmacology, 137*(1), 371-381. doi:10.1016/j.jep.2011.05.040 accessed 4/21/2017

Maas, M., Hensel, A., Costa, F. B., Brun, R., Kaiser, M., & Schmidt, T. J. (2011). An unusual dimeric guaianolide with antiprotozoal activity and further sesquiterpene lactones from Eupatorium perfoliatum. *Phytochemistry, 72*(7), 635-644. doi:10.1016/j.phytochem.2011.01.025, accessed 4/21/2017

Habtemariam, S., & Macpherson, A. M. (2000). Cytotoxicity and antibacterial activity of ethanol extract from leaves of a herbal drug, Boneset (Eupatorium perfoliatum). *Phytotherapy Research, 14*(7), 575-577. doi:10.1002/1099-1573(200011)14:7<575::aid-ptr652>3.0.co;2-1 accessed 4/21/2017

Elsässer-Beile, U., Willenbacher, W., Bartsch, H., Gallati, H., Mönting, J. S., & Von Kleist, S. (1996). Cytokine production in leukocyte cultures during therapy with echinacea extract. *Journal of Clinical Laboratory Analysis, 10*(6), 441-445. doi:10.1002/(sici)1098-2825(1996)10:6<441::aid-jcla22>3.3.co;2-y, accessed 4/21/2017

Wagner, H., Kraus, S., & Jurcic, K. (1999). Search for potent immunostimulating agents from plants and other natural sources. *Immunomodulatory Agents from Plants*, 1-39. doi:10.1007/978-3-0348-8763-2_1accessed 4/21/2017

[A controlled clinical trial for testing the efficacy of the homeopathic drug eupatorium perfoliatum D2 in the treatment of common cold (author's tr... - PubMed - NCBI. (n.d.). Retrieved from https://www.ncbi.nlm.nih.gov/pubmed/7195723, accessed 4/21/2017

Boneset Herb Benefits. (n.d.). Retrieved from
http://www.anniesremedy.com/eupatorium-perfoliatum-boneset.php,   accessed
        4/21/2017

Boneset Uses, Benefits & Side Effects - Drugs.com Herbal Database. (n.d.).
Retrieved from https://www.drugs.com/npc/boneset.html, accessed 4/21/2017

BONESET: Uses, Side Effects, Interactions, and Warnings - WebMD. (n.d.).
Retrieved   from   http://www.webmd.com/vitaminssupplements/ingredientmono-
        594\BONESET.aspx?activeIngredientId=594&activeIngredientName=B
        ONESET&source=0, accessed 4/21/2017

Eupatorium perfoliatum (Boneset) medicinal uses and photos. (n.d.). Retrieved from
        http://www.homeremediess.com/eupatorium-perfoliatum-boneset-
        medicinal-uses/, accessed 4/21/2017

A   Modern   Herbal | Boneset.   (n.d.).   Retrieved   from
        http://www.botanical.com/botanical/mgmh/b/bonese65.html,   accessed
        4/21/2017

Richard   Whelan   ~   Medical   Herbalist   ~   Boneset.   (n.d.).   Retrieved   from
        http://www.rjwhelan.co.nz/herbs%20A-Z/boneset.html,   accessed
        4/21/2017

The world's top news source on natural health - NaturalNews.com. (n.d.). Retrieved
        from
        http://www.naturalnews.com/032076_Boneset_fever_remedies.html,
        accessed 4/21/2017

Elderberry

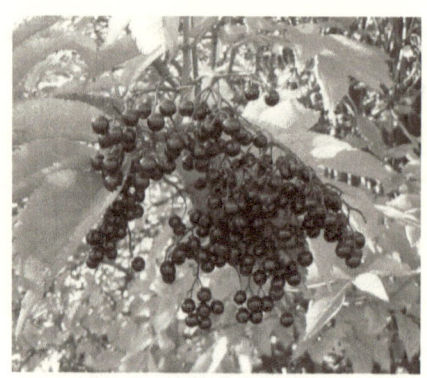

When I was a kid, my uncle would drink elderberry wine shots to nip a cold or respiratory illness in the bud. The shrub-like trees grow quickly in my geographic area; the berries produce a great juice. Homemade wines from the liquid are something of a treat, as well.

Besides being slightly yummy, Elderberries have long been used for ailments of the respiratory tract. It is commonly found in Europe and North America. Here, it grows in the areas next to small streams and drainage ditches. It sometimes appears to be more of a thick bush than a tree, but can get about 30 feet tall.

The herbal literature from the 1800s and earlier reflect its use. The United States Food & Drug Administration lists elderberry as GRAS (generally recognized as safe). It has been made into many commercial preparations available in many health foods and big box stores.

Recent studies show elderberry to be of great value when stimulating the immune system. In combination with Astragalus and Echinacea, it can boost the levels of interferon produced by *Lactobacillus* bacteria. Other studies show it, as well as the pectin from the elderflowers, stimulate the production of macrophages.

I find sipping on the wine, or some that have gone to brandy, can quiet a cough and offer sore throat relief. Elderberry is also the most natural remedy to get my kids to use. The taste of elderberry syrup or chewable products is delightful. I use them for my kids and they often think I am giving them candy. So, beware, you may have to hide your elderberry products, so your children do not eat or drink all of it.

Sources:

three benefits of black elderberry syrup for our immune system. (n.d.). Retrieved from http://www.ethnoherbalist.com/benefits-of-elderberry-black-elderberry-syrup-for-colds/

7 Surprising Elderberries Benefits | Organic Facts. (n.d.). Retrieved from https://www.organicfacts.net/health-benefits/fruit/elderberries.html

Elderberry Benefits & Information (Sambucus Nigra). (n.d.). Retrieved from http://www.herbwisdom.com/herb-elderberry.html

Elderberry Benefits & Uses, Including Cold & Flu Treatment - Dr. Axe. (n.d.). Retrieved from https://draxe.com/elderberry/

Elderberry Syrup Benefits | LIVESTRONG.COM. (n.d.). Retrieved from http://www.livestrong.com/article/115535-elderberry-syrup-benefits/

Elderberry | University of Maryland Medical Center. (n.d.). Retrieved from http://www.umm.edu/health/medical/altmed/herb/elderberry

ELDERBERRY: Uses, Side Effects, Interactions, and Warnings - WebMD. (n.d.). Retrieved from http://www.webmd.com/vitamins-supplements/ingredientmono-434-elderberry.aspx?activeingredientid=434&activeingredientname=elderberry

Frøkiær, H., Henningsen, L., Metzdorff, S. B., Weiss, G., Roller, M., Flanagan, J., ... Ibarra, A. (2012). Astragalus Root and Elderberry Fruit Extracts Enhance the IFN-β Stimulatory Effects of Lactobacillus acidophilus in Murine-Derived Dendritic Cells. *PLoS ONE, 7*(10), e47878. doi:10.1371/journal.pone.0047878

The great health benefits of elderberry - NaturalNews.com. (n.d.). Retrieved from http://www.naturalnews.com/043430_elderberry_natural_antivirals_health_benefits.html

Porter, R. S., & Bode, R. F. (2017). A Review of the Antiviral Properties of Black Elder (Sambucus nigraL.) Products. *Phytotherapy Research, 31*(4), 533-554. doi:10.1002/ptr.5782

What Are Elderberries Good For? - Mercola.com. (n.d.). Retrieved from http://foodfacts.mercola.com/elderberries.html

photo credit:

Williams, T.Retrieved from http://www.freeimages.com/photo/elderberry-delight-1326492, 5/18/2017

Astragalus

*I*f you haven't noticed, a lot of these herbs I have been highlighting increase the activity of individual immune cells known as killer cells and stimulate the production of antibodies. Astragalus is no different. It, too, beefs up the body's production of these cells. These cells, in turn, go after the germs just as a trained attack dog would go after an unauthorized intruder in your home.

Considered an adaptogen (meaning it aids the body "adapt to stresses"), Astragalus seems to offer a deeper level of immune support than Echinacea. Sometimes it can be found in formulas together because of the slightly different mechanisms each may trigger. Astragalus seems to sound an alarm which instantly awakens dormant immune cells from a sort of "sleep state" to jump into action, just like that guard dog I mentioned above.

There are studies that show Astragalus has a tonifying effect on the heart muscle. The Chinese have traditionally thought of Astragalus as a supportive immune booster for those types of people who always seem to be in a state of fatigue. It is also suggested by some Chinese herbalists for recovery from illness because of this. It seems to support the body's energy levels. I, personally, like to think of this as a go-to herb for those people who never quite seem to kick an illness. You know, the ones that go from cold to cold all winter long. Yeah, those are the people for which I suggest Astragalus.

So while Traditional Chinese Medicine considers Astragalus to be a spleen strengthener and a powerhouse to augment qi (pronounced Chi), you can think of it as the support for the bone tiredness sometimes associated with prolonged illness.

This herb has been researched in the laboratory and real-life applications. It has shown promise in all cases. Researchers have applied knowledge of this herbal to pigs, fish, and humans to demonstrate its abilities to stimulate immune responses and exert a heart-protective action. It even has been shown to increase growth factors and immune factors in pig colostrum, which may indicate it can do the same in human breast milk. I breastfed four sons. I know just how tired a new mother can be. The immune system can be extremely worn down when trying to keep up with the demands of a hungry newborn and the rest that life can hand you.

When you find Astragalus in a health food store or online, usually it will be the root and in a few different forms. The dried sliced source is the most popular form in Chinese herb shops. It can also be available as a powder. It is used in teas and has a pretty pleasant taste. Tinctures can be found in alcohol bases (usually ethanol, which you can think of as 100 proof vodka, basically). Capsules are available for the ease of use, too.

Liquid forms, such as teas, have been known to be used in amounts of 9 grams to 30 grams with no known ill side effects. According to my research, there is no toxicity associated with ingesting large amounts. Of course, each person is different and I urge anyone who uses any herbal remedies to monitor your health closely. This IS a direct immune system stimulator. Therefore, DO NOT USE IF YOU HAVE BEEN DIAGNOSED WITH AN AUTOIMMUNE DISORDER (examples include, but are not limited to Chrone's, Hashimoto Thyroiditis, Multiple Sclerosis, Lupus, etc.).

Huang Qi is the name Astragalus is known by in Traditional Chinese Medicine. The Latin classification name is *Astragalus membraneous*. These other names for the plant can be helpful as some herb labels use multiple names for the same plant.

Sources:

10 Proven Benefits of Astragalus Root (#4 Is Vital) - Dr. Axe. (n.d.). Retrieved from https://draxe.com/astragalus/

Abdullahi, A. Y., Kallon, S., Yu, X., Zhang, Y., & Li, G. (2016). Vaccination with Astragalus and Ginseng Polysaccharides Improves Immune Response of Chickens against H5N1 Avian Influenza Virus. *BioMed Research International, 2016*, 1-8. doi:10.1155/2016/1510264

Astragalus - DrWeil.com. (n.d.). Retrieved from https://www.drweil.com/vitamins-supplements-herbs/herbs/astragalus/

Astragalus Is The Safe and Effective Immune System Enhancer! | Smart
    Publications.   (n.d.).   Retrieved   from   http://www.smart-
    publications.com/articles/astragalus-is-the-safe-and-effective-immune-
    system-enhancer

Astragalus "super herb" protects, supports immune system function -
    NaturalNews.com.   (n.d.).   Retrieved   from
    http://www.naturalnews.com/027223_ASTRAGALUS_immune_system.
    html

Astragalus | University of Maryland Medical Center. (n.d.). Retrieved from
    http://www.umm.edu/health/medical/altmed/herb/astragalus

Astragalus: The Immune Warrior | alive. (n.d.). Retrieved from
    http://www.alive.com/health/astragalus-the-immune-warrior/

Block, K. I., & Mead, M. N. (2003). Immune System Effects of Echinacea, Ginseng,
    and Astragalus: A Review. *Integrative Cancer Therapies, 2*(3), 247-267.
    doi:10.1177/1534735403256419

Effect of two Chinese herbs (Astragalus radix and Scutellaria radix) on non-specific
    immune response of tilapia, Oreochromis niloticus - ScienceDirect.
    (n.d.).   Retrieved   from
    http://www.sciencedirect.com/science/article/pii/S0044848605004229

Elabd, H., Wang, H., Shaheen, A., Yao, H., & Abbass, A. (2016). Feeding
    Glycyrrhiza glabra (licorice) and Astragalus membranaceus (AM) alters
    innate immune and physiological responses in yellow perch (Perca
    flavescens). *Fish & Shellfish Immunology, 54,* 374-384.
    doi:10.1016/j.fsi.2016.04.024

Global protein expression analysis of molecular markers of DS-1-47, a component
    of implantation-promoting traditional Chinese medicine. - PubMed -
    NCBI.   (n.d.).   Retrieved   from
    https://www.ncbi.nlm.nih.gov/pubmed/27924510

Lai, X., Xia, W., Wei, J., & Ding, X. (2017). Therapeutic Effect of Astragalus
    Polysaccharides on Hepatocellular Carcinoma H22-Bearing Mice. *Dose-
    Response, 15*(1), 155932581668518. doi:10.1177/1559325816685182

Lan, R. X., Park, J. W., Lee, D. W., & Kim, I. H. (2016). Effects of astragalus
    membranaceus,Codonopsis pilosulaand allicin mixture on growth
    performance, nutrient digestibility, fecal microbial shedding, immune
    response and meat quality in finishing pigs. *Journal of Animal
    Physiology and Animal Nutrition.* doi:10.1111/jpn.12625

Li, J., Huang, L., Wang, S., Yao, Y., & Zhang, Z. (2016). Astragaloside IV
    attenuates inflammatory reaction via activating immune function of
    regulatory T-cells inhibited by HMGB1 in mice. *Pharmaceutical
    Biology, 54*(12), 3217-3225. doi:10.1080/13880209.2016.1216133

The Many Benefits of the Immune-Boosting Root Astragalus | Natural Society.
    (n.d.). Retrieved from http://naturalsociety.com/health-benefits-of-
    astragalus-boost-immune-system/

Shao, B., Xu, W., Dai, H., Tu, P., Li, Z., & Gao, X. (2004). A study on the immune
    receptors for polysaccharides from the roots of Astragalus
    membranaceus, a Chinese medicinal herb. *Biochemical and Biophysical
    Research   Communications, 320*(4),   1103-1111.
    doi:10.1016/j.bbrc.2004.06.065

Su, G., Chen, X., Liu, Z., Yang, L., Zhang, L., Stålsby Lundborg, C., ... Liu, X. (2015). Oral Astragalus (Huang qi) for preventing frequent episodes of acute respiratory tract infection in children. *Cochrane Database of Systematic Reviews*. doi:10.1002/14651858.cd011958

Tan, L., Wei, T., Yuan, A., He, J., Liu, J., Xu, D., & Yang, Q. (2017). Dietary Supplementation of Astragalus Polysaccharides Enhanced Immune Components and Growth Factors EGF and IGF-1 in Sow Colostrum. *Journal of Immunology Research, 2017*, 1-6. doi:10.1155/2017/9253208

Yu, Z., Guo, F., Guo, Y., Zhang, Z., Wu, F., & Luo, X. (2017). Optimization and evaluation of Astragalus polysaccharide injectable thermoresponsive in-situ gels. *PLOS ONE, 12*(3), e0173949. doi:10.1371/journal.pone.0173949

Zhou, L., Liu, Z., Wang, Z., Yu, S., Long, T., Zhou, X., & Bao, Y. (2017). Astragalus polysaccharides exert immunomodulatory effects via TLR4-mediated MyD88-dependent signaling pathway in vitro and in vivo. *Scientific Reports, 7*, 44822. doi:10.1038/srep44822

Zhu, N., Lv, X., Wang, Y., Li, J., Liu, Y., Lu, W., ... Zhang, L. W. (2016). Comparison of immunoregulatory effects of polysaccharides from three natural herbs and cellular uptake in dendritic cells. *International Journal of Biological Macromolecules, 93*, 940-951. doi:10.1016/j.ijbiomac.2016.09.064

Cat's Claw

*U*na de Gato. The claw of the cat. *Uncaria tomentosa* is a vining plant found in the Peruvian rainforest. The name is derived from the tiny nails that protrude from the vine, which resemble feline's claws. It is also an immune boosting herb which has been extensively studied since the 1970s.

While most people have never heard of this herb, it has been looked at as one potential plant to aid in the fight against immune system impairment. Much research in Peru, Austria, Germany, England, Hungary and other locations have investigated its strong abilities to stimulate the immune system.

The bark of the roots of Cat's Claw holds something called Isopteropodin. This is an alkaloid. Alkaloids are bitter to the taste. This particular one seems to increase the body's immune response when ingested and behaves as an antioxidant. This means it counteracts some of the effects of toxins, pollution, age, stress, and so forth upon the cells of the human body. How freaking awesome that?

The alkaloids contained in Cat's Claw are so savage that they enhance the ability of the human body's white blood cells to engulf pathogens to destroy them.

Cat's Claw is said to be immune-regulatory. That means unlike some other immune stimulators, it possesses the ability to regulate the immune system function. If it is over-active, Cat's Claw can dial it down. If the resistance is under-active, Cat's Claw can kick it in the pants to get those immune cells functioning. This means Cat's Claw has been looked at for its ability to aid issues with the gut and bowel. Correctly, it shows promise in helping those individuals suffering from irritable bowel, chrone's, and leaky gut as well as some other gut and bowel issues.

It also has been shown to function as an excellent anti-inflammatory herb. Much research has been devoted to its uses to enhance pain-free movement, reduce pain associated with gout, and overall anti-inflammatory type actions.

The most bad-ass part about Cat's Claw is that it has been shown to inhibit the growth and spread (proliferation) of some types of cancer. This makes this rainforest gem a wonder herb in my book.

Cat's Claw is used as a decoction or infusion (tea), extract, and encapsulated. Most research indicates using up to 350 mg of this herb per day. Some research suggests using Cat's Claw which has been standardized to contain 8% carboxy alkyl esters for maximum anti-inflammatory action.

I have been very open about my battle against specific gut issues. I have a very touchy gut. At any moment, odd diet combinations or varying levels of high stress and anxiety may touch off periods of constipation or diarrhea. Truthfully, I really could not tell you which freaking one is worse. They both piss me off. I just want to poop like a "normal" person.

Anyhow, upon the suggestion of a friend, I used some Cat's Claw to deal with the oddball bloaty-swollen feeling accompanying one of these spells. It worked. I do not use it regularly, but when things get out of hand, it's there for me. I have the added benefit of knowing if there is a touch of some strange bad-guy infection causing this flare up, It will boost up my good guys to take care of the job.

While research has shown little adverse side effects of large doses of Cat's Claw, it _**is**_ _**CONTRAINDICATED IN PREGNANCY**_ as it could induce a miscarriage. Also note: _Uncaria guianensis_ is also Cat's Claw. This particular type is better for wound healing, according to sources. Be sure to get the _Uncaria tomentosa_ or the immune regulatory effects. Despite its immunoregulatory functions, it is not suggested that people with autoimmune disorders like Multiple Sclerosis or Lupus uses Cat's Claw for any prolonged period.

Sources:

8 Cat's Claw Benefits for Immunity, Digestion & Chronic Disease - Dr. Axe. (n.d.). Retrieved from https://draxe.com/cats-claw/

Cats Claw Benefits & Information (Uncaria Tomentosa). (n.d.). Retrieved from http://www.herbwisdom.com/herb-cats-claw.html

Cat's Claw | Life Extension Magazine. (n.d.). Retrieved from http://www.lifeextension.com/magazine/2007/3/nu_catsclaw/page-01

Cat's Claw | Life Extension Magazine. (n.d.). Retrieved from http://www.lifeextension.com/magazine/2007/3/nu_catsclaw/page-01

Cat's claw | University of Maryland Medical Center. (n.d.). Retrieved from http://www.umm.edu/health/medical/altmed/herb/cats-claw

Cat's Claw. (n.d.). Retrieved from https://www.drugs.com/cdi/cat-s-claw.html

Discover the incredible healing properties of Cat's Claw - NaturalNews.com. (n.d.). Retrieved from http://www.naturalnews.com/032917_cats_claw_herb.html

Domingues, A., Sartori, A., Golim, M. A., Valente, L. M., Da Rosa, L. C., Ishikawa, L. L., ... Viero, R. M. (2011). Prevention of experimental diabetes by Uncaria tomentosa extract: Th2 polarization, regulatory T cell preservation or both? *Journal of Ethnopharmacology, 137*(1), 635-642. doi:10.1016/j.jep.2011.06.021

Eberlin, S., Dos Santos, L. M., & Queiroz, M. L. (2005). Uncaria tomentosa extract increases the number of myeloid progenitor cells in the bone marrow of mice infected with Listeria monocytogenes. *International Immunopharmacology, 5*(7-8), 1235-1246. doi:10.1016/j.intimp.2005.03.001

Erowele, G. I., & Kalejaiye, A. O. (2009). Pharmacology and therapeutic uses of cat's claw. *American Journal of Health-System Pharmacy, 66*(11), 992-995. doi:10.2146/ajhp080443

Pero, R., Amiri, A., Sheng, Y., Welther, M., & Rich, M. (2005). Formulation and in vitro/in vivo evaluation of combining DNA repair and immune enhancing nutritional supplements. *Phytomedicine, 12*(4), 255-263. doi:10.1016/j.phymed.2004.01.008

Uncaria tomentosa alkaloidal fraction reduces paracellular permeability, IL-8 and NS1 production on human microvascular endothelial cells infected ... - PubMed - NCBI. (n.d.). Retrieved from https://www.ncbi.nlm.nih.gov/pubmed/24427938

Uses and benefits of Cat's Claw. (n.d.). Retrieved from http://all-natural.com/natural-remedies/catsclaw/

Yunis-Aguinaga, J., Claudiano, G. S., Marcusso, P. F., Manrique, W. G., De Moraes, J. R., De Moraes, F. R., & Fernandes, J. B. (2015). Uncaria tomentosa increases growth and immune activity in Oreochromis niloticus challenged with Streptococcus agalactiae. *Fish & Shellfish Immunology, 47*(1), 630-638. doi:10.1016/j.fsi.2015.09.051

Licorice Root

So many people gag and gross out over black jelly beans that they never give this herb a fair try. I am one of those weirdos that happens to like black jelly beans, but in reality, those are not made with actual licorice. Often, they are made with an herbal extract from anise (also useful, but not what we are talking about here).

Real licorice comes from a root of a plant which grows in eastern Europe and parts of India. It is a part of the legume family. The sap contained in the factory is a thick, syrupy consistency and has a mild, sweet flavor. *Glycyrrhiza glabra* is a bush that grows to about five feet and comes back every year (a perennial).

Licorice is often in oral preparations for a sore throat and upper respiratory complaints. In Ayurveda (Traditional Indian Medicine) it is called Yashtimadhu, which translates as sweet stem or stalk. It is said to be about fifty times sweeter than sugar. I am not a huge fan of super sweet flavors, so straight licorice is a bit overwhelming for my pallet.

It is high in various antioxidants (flavonoids, saponins, sterols, choline, coumarins, lignins, triterpenoids). It contains amino acids (asparagine being one), gums, biotin, folic acid, inositol, lecithin, estrogenic substances, pantothenic acid, para-aminobenzoic acid, phosphorous, certain types of terpenes, and vitamins B1, B2, B3, B6, and E. It has been shown to contain estrogenic like substances.

Recent research has shown licorice has an immunomodulatory effect. This means it has more of a regulatory function over the immune cells than one of just stimulatory action. Mainly, research has pointed to its regulatory effects on the macrophages. Macrophages are the "big eaters" of the white blood cells (literally, that's how macrophage translates). They can morph into various shapes, engulph "foreign invaders" and then they kind of "wear" the chemical markers of the bad guy it ate on its outside to provide a warning for other cells (this is the boosting of interferon). This produces what is called non-specific immunity. Recent studies have shown it to be useful in orthodontal diseases, including candidiasis (yeast overgrowth, specifically oral overgrowth in this study). Other studies also point to its ability to inhibit cells from being subject to candida yeast infection.

It seems to be anti-allergenic. In studies, it has been shown to reduce rhinitis (running nose), itchy eyes, and other symptoms often associated with respiratory allergies. Some suggest that this is due to licorice being able to keep the adrenal hormone, cortisol, in check. There's research showing it to be promising for relaxing bronchial spasms.

It is considered protectionary for the liver. Because of this protectionary function, those people taking medications which metabolize in the liver may want to steer clear of using licorice. This would include statins and other prescription medications. If you are currently using prescription medications and want to know if your meds are broken down in the liver, ask your pharmacist. They are happy to help you. Some Traditional Chinese Medicine remedies are in tiny balls (pills or tablets) consisting of powdered herbs mixed in a licorice base. You really need to pay attention to supplement labels, and it is good to be on a conversational level with your pharmacist.

Currently, licorice is being investigated for use in HIV, influenza, and various types of hepatitis. It is indeed a natural warrior in this class as it helps to regulate the immune cells impaired by these medically diagnosed diseases.

I like to use licorice as a tea when dealing with right issues of the mouth and throat. It can be quite yummy, and I have never needed any additional sweetener for it. In my experience, it soothes the dry hacking coughs and relaxes the tight chest feeling I have often experienced throughout the Ohio harvest season.

Also, licorice has been shown to inhibit the growth of gram-negative bacteria, most notably *Helicobacter pylori*. Therefore, it is found in many stomachs comforting herbal blends. Some people have tried these combinations before turning to synthetic medications that turn off the proton pumps (acid-making cells) in the stomach with some success.

Licorice is not without contraindications. The maximum dose suggested by some sources is six (6) grams for a person weighing 130 pounds. Please exercise discretion when using it. Side effects to watch for are chronic fatigue, high blood pressure, edema (swelling), and low potassium levels. This would indicate you are using too much licorice.

DO NOT USE LICORICE IF YOU HAVE HIGH BLOOD PRESSURE or if you are currently on prescription blood pressure medications, digoxin, prescription corticosteroids, prescription and some over-the-counter diuretics (water pills), statins or any medication broken down (changed) in the liver.

sources:

Messier, C., Epifano, F., Genovese, S., & Grenier, D. (2011). Licorice and its potential beneficial effects in common oro-dental diseases. *Oral Diseases,18*(1), 32-39. doi:10.1111/j.1601-0825.2011.01842.x

Li, J., Tu, Y., Tong, L., Zhang, W., Zheng, J., & Wei, Q. (2010). Immunosuppressive activity on the murine immune responses of glycerol fromGlycyrrhiza uralensisvia inhibition of calcineurin activity. *Pharmaceutical Biology,48*(10), 1177-1184. doi:10.3109/13880200903573169

Lee, J. Y., Lee, J. H., Park, J. H., Kim, S. Y., Choi, J. Y., Lee, S. H., . . . Han, Y. (2009, May). Liquiritigenin, a licorice flavonoid, helps mice resist disseminated candidiasis due to Candida albicans by a Th1 immune response, whereas liquidity, its glycoside form, does not. Retrieved October 13, 2017, from https://www.ncbi.nlm.nih.gov/pubmed/19264152

Cheng, A., Wan, F., Wang, J., Jin, Z., & Xu, X. (2008, January). Macrophage immunomodulatory activity of polysaccharides isolated from Glycyrrhiza uralensis Fish. Retrieved October 13, 2017, from https://www.ncbi.nlm.nih.gov/pubmed/18068099

Licorice Root Benefits & Information (Glycyrrhiza Glabra). (n.d.). Retrieved October 13, 2017, from http://www.herbwisdom.com/herb-licorice-root.html

Boldt, E. (2017, August 09). Licorice Root Benefits Adrenal Fatigue & Leaky Gut. Retrieved October 13, 2017, from https://draxe.com/licorice-root/

Irani, M., Sarmadi, M., Bernard, F., Pour, G. H., & Bazarnov, H. S. (2010). Leaves Antimicrobial Activity of *Glycyrrhiza glabr*Lous. Retrieved October 13, 2017, from https://www.ncbi.nlm.nih.gov/pmc/articles/PMC3870067/

(n.d.). Retrieved October 18, 2017, from http://www.medindia.net/alternativemedicine/liquorice-yashtimadhu.asp

Mandal, M. D. (2014, January 14). What is a Macrophage? Retrieved October 18, 2017, from https://www.news-medical.net/life-sciences/What-is-a-Macrophage.aspx

St. John's Wort

*T*he classification name for this plant is *Hypericum perforatum*, and it has received a ton of coverage through the years as it is studied for its ability to be of assistance in mild bouts of depression. However, it also has a lesser-known history of being used when respiratory ailments are present.

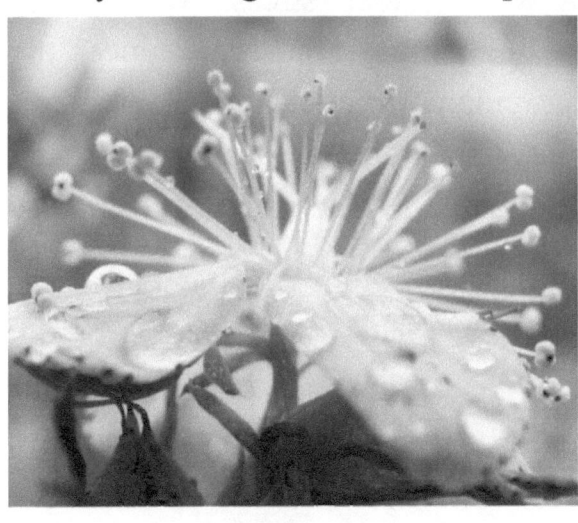

Also known as Klamath Weed or Goat Weed, it has been confirmed to be in use since about the first century AD by the writings of Greek herbalist Dioskourides. It is said the name of St. John's Wort was bestowed upon it by early Christians because it blooms near the feast day of John the Baptist.

While the mechanisms of how this plant works are still being investigated, many hypotheses are suggesting that its ability to help regulate stress may also have a beneficial result for the immune system. Decreases in corticosteroid levels have been found when it is used in studies. Corticosteroids are produced when the body is under stress. While they decrease swelling, they tend to reduce the activity of individual immune cells. They can function as a "fail-safe" measure to keep immune reactions in check, or they can suppress it into ineffectiveness.

One study suggests its antispasmodic effects on the gastrointestinal and respiratory tracts being due to an inhibitory effect on calcium influx and phosphodiesterase. It also has been shown to exert a protection to the endothelial cells in lungs of rats when it is exposed to a particular herbicide. It also seems it has been found to help increase the number of regulatory T (T reg) cells in the spleen in laboratory studies. T reg cells can suppress the activity of other immune cells. The authors of this research hinted at this being a possible bonus when seeking methods for the regulation of autoimmune disorders.

My personal experience with it was during a bought of the gut "flu." The term "gut flu" is a misnomer, as usually, the symptoms that come to mind are actually from mild bacterial infections. To be clear, I was suffering from gut-wrenching diarrhea and nausea and vomiting. A local herbalist I know instructed me to put St. Johns Wort extract (labeled as Klammath Weed) into my belly button. While I was in my early 20's at the time and I thought she was batshit crazy, I did it. No lie, the extract seemed to soak in, and the gut pains subsided for a moment. Each time I used the extract in this manner, the frequency of the pain became less and less, until it had passed.

Of all the studies I read about this herb and its use associated with immunological studies, one did discuss negative results when used with mice infected with H1N1 (swine flu). In this study, the mice experienced increased swelling of lung membranes, etc. This is something to keep in mind. *It probably would not be my first choice in a severe illness displaying viral flu-like symptoms.*

St. John's Wort does have unique **contraindications. It is not advised for use if you are taking any of the following types of pharmaceuticals: anticancer agents; anti-HIV agents; anti-inflammatory agents (including ibuprofen); antimicrobial/antibiotic agents; cardiovascular drugs (blood pressure and blood thinning meds); central nervous system agents (SSRIs and other neurotransmitter meds); hypoglycemic agents; immuno-modulating agents; oral contraceptives; proton pump inhibitor (Nexium and the like); respiratory system agent; and statins.

Sources:

[Effect of Hypericum perforatum on preventing acute injury of rat pulmonary microvascular endothelial cells induced by paraquat]. - PubMed - NCBI. (n.d.). Retrieved from https://www.ncbi.nlm.nih.gov/pubmed/16761427

Barnes, J., Anderson, L. A., & Phillipson, J. D. (2001). St John's wort (Hypericum perforatumL.): a review of its chemistry, pharmacology and clinical properties. *Journal of Pharmacy and Pharmacology*, *53*(5), 583-600. doi:10.1211/0022357011775910

Corticosteroids & Prednisone Information | Cleveland Clinic. (n.d.). Retrieved from http://my.clevelandclinic.org/health/articles/corticosteroids

Di, Y., Li, C., Xue, C., & Zhou, S. (2008). Clinical Drugs that Interact with St. Johns Wort and implication in Drug Development. *Current Pharmaceutical Design*, *14*(17), 1723-1742. doi:10.2174/138161208784746798

Gilani, A. H., Khan, A., Subhan, F., & Khan, M. (2005). Antispasmodic and bronchodilator activities of St John's wort are putatively mediated through dual inhibition of calcium influx and phosphodiesterase. *Fundamental and Clinical Pharmacology*, *19*(6), 695-705. doi:10.1111/j.1472-8206.2005.00378.x

Grundmann, O., Lv, Y., Kelber, O., & Butterweck, V. (2010). Mechanism of St. John's wort extract (STW3-VI) during chronic restraint stress is mediated by the interrelationship of the immune, oxidative defense, and neuroendocrine system. *Neuropharmacology*, *58*(4-5), 767-773. doi:10.1016/j.neuropharm.2009.12.014

History and therapeutic properties of Hypericum Perforatum from antiquity until today. - PubMed - NCBI. (n.d.). Retrieved from https://www.ncbi.nlm.nih.gov/pubmed/21914616

History and therapeutic properties of Hypericum Perforatum from antiquity until today. - PubMed - NCBI. (n.d.). Retrieved from https://www.ncbi.nlm.nih.gov/pubmed/21914616

Immunity: plants as effective mediators. - PubMed - NCBI. (n.d.). Retrieved from https://www.ncbi.nlm.nih.gov/pubmed/24564587

The immuno-regulatory impact of orally-administered Hypericum perforatum extracts on Balb/C mice inoculated with H1n1 influenza A virus. - PubMed - NCBI. (n.d.). Retrieved from https://www.ncbi.nlm.nih.gov/pubmed/24098792

Nandakumar, S., Miller, C. W., & Kumaraguru, U. (2009). T regulatory cells: an overview and intervention techniques to modulate allergy outcome. *Clinical and Molecular Allergy*, *7*(1), 5. doi:10.1186/1476-7961-7-5

Nosratabadi, R., Rastin, M., Sankian, M., Haghmorad, D., Tabasi, N., Zamani, S., … Mahmoudi, M. (2015). St. John's wort and its component hyperforin alleviate experimental autoimmune encephalomyelitis through expansion of regulatory T-cells. *Journal of Immunotoxicology*, *13*(3), 364-374. doi:10.3109/1547691x.2015.1101512

73

Perfume, M. (2001). Effects of a methanolic extract and a hyperforin-enriched CO_2 extract of Hypericum perforatum on alcohol intake in rats. *Alcohol and Alcoholism, 36*(3), 199-206. doi:10.1093/alcalc/36.3.199

Sellers, H. S., Villegas, P. N., El-Attrache, J., Kapczynski, D. R., & Brown, C. C. (2001). Detection of Infectious Bursal Disease Virus in Experimentally Infected Chickens by in situ Hybridization. *Avian Diseases, 45*(1), 26. doi:10.2307/1593008

photo credit:

Michaela Kobyakov, **http://www.freeimages.com/photo/st-john-s-wort-1148375,** 5/18/2017

Appendix

Silver Sol

Colloidal silver has had a wild ride as a "miracle cure" (I use that term very loosely). However, the silver particles in most colloidal preparations of colloidal silver can be too large for the body's waste systems to handle. While silver is not generally thought to be toxic to regular healthy cells, per se, they can become trapped in the body and turn a person an odd bluish grey color.

In the early 1900's the term "blue blood" referred to wealthy people turning this particular hue due to the cheap silver plating of eating utensils at the time. Acids in the food and saliva would cause a person to digest quantities of silver. These particles were too large to be filtered out of the bloodstream by the kidneys, and a person would be blue (a condition known as Agyrya).

After the dawn of home-made colloidal silver machines, the concern over silver toxicity became heightened once again. More recently, other forms of silver have come into use, as well.

There is much debate on the topic of using silver for the immune system. Since it is not an herb and must be highly processed to be used, I included this substance under the Appendix section. Silver is technically a naturally occurring element. It is used by the body in minute trace amounts every single day. However, when looking at using a silver product for immune system support use, a person would use much more than what is taken in by consuming a regular diet. This is when I find research on silver solutions helpful.

The silver solution, also known as a Silver Sol, is a particle consisting of silver atoms and oxygen atoms and is much different than its predecessor, colloidal silver. Silver sol has particles which are much smaller than colloidal silver. It has been studied for human safety and has yielded promising results. Internal use research has shown it to increase immune cells' ability to fend off foreign invaders. It is being researched for its promise in wound care and can fight off pathogens externally. Some companies sell it in the form of a gel to be used as a hand sanitizer type of thing and even in pre-made bandages. Further research supporting its ability to sanitize skin lends, even more, evidence to use it as an external skin spritzer or spray.

Some sources suggest this type of silver may protect the body's immune cells while allowing for the demise of the unwanted invaders (viruses, bacteria, etc.). I use Silver Sol as soon as I get that tired feeling. You know the feeling: a sore throat, bone tired, groggy, achy. That is when I begin using an ounce of silver sol three to four times a day conjunction with other immune stimulating herbs and teas. I, personally, want to use every tool I have available.

Sources:

OHP, J. B. (n.d.). What is the Difference Between Colloidal Silver and a Silver Solution? Retrieved October 18, 2017, from http://blog.optimumhealthvitamins.com/what-is-the-difference-between-colloidal-silver-and-a-silver-solution

Barbasz, A., Oćwieja, M., & Barbasz, J. (2015). Cytotoxic Activity of Highly Purified Silver Nanoparticles Sol Against Cells of Human Immune System. Applied Biochemistry and Biotechnology, 176(3), 817-834. doi:10.1007/s12010-015-1613-3

Lansdown, A. B. (2004). A review of the use of silver in wound care: facts and fallacies. British Journal of Nursing, 13(Sup1). doi:10.12968/bjon.2004.13.sup1.12535

Rai, M., Deshmukh, S., Ingle, A., & Gade, A. (2012). Silver nanoparticles: the powerful nanoweapon against multidrug-resistant bacteria. Journal of Applied Microbiology, 112(5), 841-852. doi:10.1111/j.1365-2672.2012.05253.x

Kelly, E., & Stahl, J. (2013). Faculty of 1000 evaluation for Silver enhances antibiotic activity against gram-negative bacteria. *F1000 - Post-publication peer review of the biomedical literature*. doi:10.3410/f.718023276.793480349

Pokrowiecki, R., Zareba, T., Mielczarek, A., Opalińska, A., Wojnarowicz, J., Majkowski, M., . . . Tyski, S. (n.d.). [Evaluation of biocidal properties of silver nanoparticles against cariogenic bacteria]. Retrieved October 18, 2017, from https://www.ncbi.nlm.nih.gov/pubmed/24432559

Dr. Edward Group DC, NP, DACBN, DCBCN, DABFM. (2017, June 16). Do You Know These 3 Types of Colloidal Silver? Retrieved October 18, 2017, from https://www.globalhealingcenter.com/natural-health/3-types-silver/

Conclusion

Modern medicine is a beautiful and miraculous thing with monumental discoveries every single day. However, there is so much each of us can do to keep ourselves as healthy as possible so that the medical community is there to deal with the big stuff. To me it is clear. We owe it to ourselves and those around us to utilize herbal and natural wisdom whenever we can.

Maintaining our health is ultimately our responsibility. Over the years, it has become fashionable to figuratively sign our health responsibilities over to medical personnel. This isn't fair to ourselves, and it's not appropriate to stick the medical staff with the sole burden. Each of us is responsible for taking care of the vehicle we live in each day: our bodies.

Our bodies are natural, living organisms which benefit significantly from being fed natural, living foods. It only seems fitting that we use native plants (herbs) and supplements to help keep ourselves healthy. I am hoping this little herbal might aid you in finding a Natural Warrior to aid in your immune battles.